LEMONS
are a
GIRL'S BEST FRIEND

Conceived and produced by Elwin Street Productions Limited
14 Clerkenwell Green
London, EC1R 0DP
elwinstreet.com

Published in the United States by Clarkson Potter/Publishers, an imprint
of the Crown Publishing Group, a division of Penguin Random House LLC,
New York.
crownpublishing.com
clarksonpotter.com

CLARKSON POTTER is a trademark and POTTER with colophon is a
registered trademark of Penguin Random House LLC.

Library of Congress Cataloging-in-Publication Data is available on request.

ISBN 978-1-5247-6305-3
Ebook ISBN 978-1-5247-6306-0
Printed in China

Illustrations by Tonwen Jones

10 9 8 7 6 5 4 3 2 1

First Edition

LEMONS
are a
GIRL'S BEST
FRIEND

Janet Hayward

Clarkson Potter/Publishers
New York

CONTENTS

INTRODUCTION

Much has been written about the importance of eating at least two servings of fruit and five servings of vegetables each day to maintain your health—but if you make an effort to include "superfruits" and "superveggies" in your diet, your skin, hair, nails, and eyes will thank you with an enviable radiant glow that the most expensive beauty products can't create.

The secret is choosing the most naturally color-rich produce. The strong pigments that give fruits and vegetables their distinctive and intense colors are actually the beneficial flavonoid compounds that have powerful antioxidant and anti-inflammatory effects. Antioxidants help neutralize free radicals in the body that can cause damage to healthy cells—so the more brightly colored fruit and vegetables in your diet, the stronger your immune system and general health will be.

As an added bonus, you'll keep your natural beauty glowing from within. These same fruits and vegetables can also work wonders when prepared and applied to your skin and body as personalized, natural beauty treatments.

This book guides you through the beautiful color spectrum of ingredients so you can choose from their amazing benefits and learn how to turn them into easy, delicious dishes and pampering beauty treatments that will ensure you look and feel like a glamazon all year round!

CHERRIES

Crisp, juicy cherries are at their best during the summer months. Mainly grown in temperate climates, these fleshy stone fruits feature in a wide range of delicious recipes, both sweet and savory.

The cherry's beautiful, deep red color comes from the powerful antioxidant anthocyanin, which acts as an anti-inflammatory and helps keep the entire body fit and healthy. Cherries are particularly rich in the minerals potassium, magnesium, and iron, as well as the B vitamins folic acid, niacin, and riboflavin. Vitamins A and C are present, too. Assisting in collagen production, these useful nutrients help maintain the elasticity of the skin, keeping it looking young and fresh.

This superfruit also contains sleep-regulating melatonin, which could suggest that cherries can contribute to a good night's rest. What better boost for all-around beauty than that?

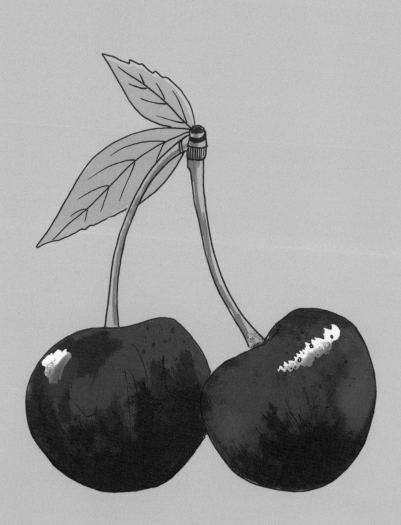

SOUR CHERRY AND MINT GRANITA

Inside: Enjoy this antioxidant- and vitamin-rich refresher to enliven your complexion.

You will need:

3 cups fresh sour cherries • 3 tablespoons coconut sugar
• 6 fresh mint leaves, plus extra for garnish • 1 cup water

To prepare:

Remove the pits from the cherries and purée in a blender with the coconut sugar, six mint leaves, and water—the mix can be smooth or chunky, depending on your preference.

Spread the purée evenly over a shallow baking sheet and freeze for 45 minutes, until solid. Return to the blender for a short blast to form the granita. Spoon into serving glasses and top each with a fresh mint leaf. Serve immediately.

CHERRY LIP TINT

Outside: Hydrate and moisturize your lips
with this pretty tinted balm.

You will need:

6 ripe, deep red cherries • 1 tablespoon coconut oil • 1 vitamin
E capsule • small glass jar with screw-top lid

To prepare:

Halve the cherries, remove the pits, and place the flesh in a
small glass bowl. Add the coconut oil and the contents of the
vitamin E capsule. Place the glass bowl over a small saucepan
of boiling water to melt the ingredients and release the juice
from the cherries. When the color of the mixture has
deepened, remove the cherry halves. Allow to cool before
pouring into the small glass jar, and storing in the refrigerator.

To use:

Apply this cherry-red tint to your lips for a hint of natural
moisturizing color.

CRANBERRIES

Native to North America and Canada, cranberries generally
grow from spring to winter, and need ample sunlight to ripen fully.
Their benefits can be enjoyed all year round, however, in
dried cranberries and juice.

This zesty super fruit's tartness is an instant indication of the
natural acidity that makes the cranberry such a great all-around
health food. The lush, red berries contain antioxidants, including
proanthocyanidins, which can offer protection from tooth decay and
inflammatory conditions. They are also a good source of vitamins
A and C, the essential B vitamins, and the minerals potassium and
manganese—a perfect cocktail for healthy skin, hair, and nails.

Bursting with phytonutrients, cranberries are often recommended
in juice form for treating urinary tract infections. This is because the
juice makes urine acidic, meaning bacteria are less likely to linger and
flourish in the bladder.

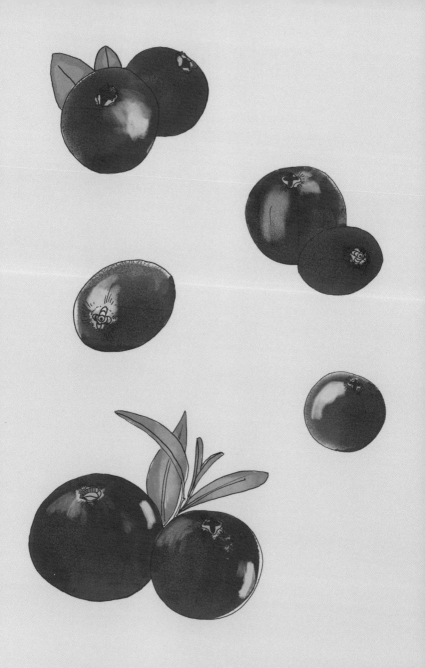

CRANBERRY-POACHED PEAR

Inside: Calm your whole body with this
light, zesty palate cleanser.

You will need:

1 ripe pear • ½ cup cranberry juice • 1 teaspoon honey

• ½ cinnamon stick • Greek yogurt (optional)

To prepare:

Peel the pear, cut into halves, and remove the core. Place in a
small saucepan with the cranberry juice, honey, and cinnamon
stick. Cover and simmer over low heat for ten minutes. Remove
the lid and simmer for an additional five minutes to reduce
the cranberry sauce.

Serve the poached pear with the cranberry sauce and a
spoonful of Greek yogurt, if desired.

CRANBERRY AND ROSE HIP TONER

Outside: Enjoy a smoother, softer face
after using this skin-toning water.

You will need:

3 tablespoons unsweetened cranberry juice • 3 tablespoons witch
hazel • 3 drops rose hip oil • small glass jar with screw-top lid

To prepare:

Carefully pour the cranberry juice, witch hazel, and rose hip
oil into the glass jar and shake vigorously to blend.

To use:

After cleansing, pour a little of the toner onto a cotton ball
and wipe gently across your face to remove any residual
makeup and dead skin cells.

GOJI BERRIES

Goji berries are native to Tibet, China, and the Himalayas, where they have been used for thousands of years for their medicinal benefits. Also known as wolfberries, these plump little superfruits boost immunity, increase alertness, and improve circulation. Fall is the season for fresh goji berries, although they can be hard to find in the West. Thankfully, they are available in dried form all year round, so you never need to run out!

Loaded with antioxidants and boasting high levels of vitamin C, goji berries are unique in that they contain all the essential amino acids and a high concentration of protein to keep the body healthy and youthful looking. These tiny, bittersweet fruits have no fewer than 21 trace minerals, including very high levels of iron, as well as selenium and zinc.

No doubt, adding a teaspoon of goji berries to your breakfast cereal or dessert will give you a glowingly healthy mind, body, and spirit!

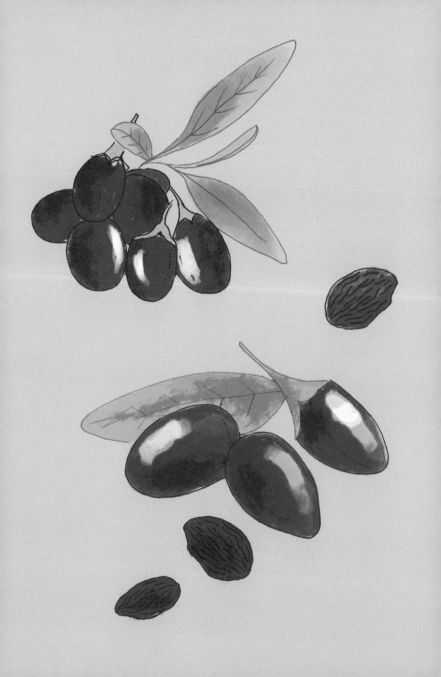

GOJI POWER SMOOTHIE

Inside: Say goodbye to mid-morning snacks with this filling, high-protein breakfast smoothie.

You will need:

1 banana • 1 kiwifruit • 3 tablespoons dried goji berries

• 1 tablespoon cacao powder • 1 cup coconut water

• 3 tablespoons yogurt

To prepare:

Peel and chop the banana and kiwi. Place in a blender and add the goji berries, cacao powder, coconut water, and yogurt. Blend together until smooth.

GOJI BERRY EXFOLIATOR

Outside: Apply this nourishing exfoliator for smooth, supple, and youthful-looking skin.

You will need:

1 tablespoon dried goji berries • ½ avocado

To prepare:

Roughly chop the goji berries and blend with the avocado to make a paste.

To use:

Gently massage onto your face and neck to exfoliate, moisturize, and enliven the skin.

POMEGRANATES

Originating in the Middle East, the Mediterranean, and northern India, the pomegranate has long played a prominent role in the history, art, and culinary traditions of these regions. With bright ruby-red juice packed into tiny seeds, this superfruit is as visually attractive as it is healthy. At its best, its flavor is a unique blend of sweet and sour, and the jewel-like seeds shine in both sweet and savory recipes.

Flourishing in fall, pomegranates bring amazing health and beauty benefits just in time for the winter months ahead. Known for their powerful antiaging and anti-inflammatory properties, these red-skinned fruits are rich in potassium, vitamin C, polyphenol, and vitamin B6. These combine to fight free-radical damage. They also boost collagen production, promoting springy, youthful-looking skin.

Drink pomegranate juice to give your immune system a boost—a glass of the richly-colored nectar offers twice the antioxidant power of the same volume of red wine or green tea.

20

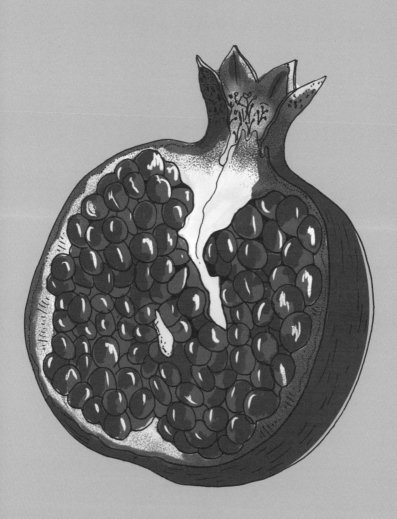

Halloumi, Orange, and Pomegranate Salad

Inside: Help combat free-radical damage with this fresh, antioxidant-rich salad.

You will need:

8 oz halloumi • 2 oranges • 1 pomegranate • ½ bunch fresh basil • olive oil • juice of ½ lemon • sea salt • black pepper

To prepare:

Cut the halloumi into eight equal slices and place under the broiler, flipping once, until golden on both sides. Peel away the skin of both oranges and divide into segments, taking care to remove the pith. Arrange the halloumi slices and orange segments on a serving plate.

Remove the seeds from the pomegranate, sprinkle over the halloumi and orange, and top with torn basil leaves. Lightly dress the salad with olive oil and lemon juice, seasoning with sea salt and black pepper to taste.

22

POMEGRANATE AND COCONUT FACIAL TREATMENT

Outside: Refresh and hydrate your skin with this highly nourishing, antiaging treatment.

You will need:

2 tablespoons pomegranate seeds • 1 tablespoon coconut oil

• 1 tablespoon honey

To prepare:

Combine all the ingredients in a bowl, mash the pomegranate seeds with a fork to release the juice, then whisk to distribute evenly throughout the mixture.

To use:

Gently massage the mixture onto your cleansed face to loosen dry skin cells. Leave it in place for five minutes to hydrate and moisturize. Rinse the mixture off using warm water and gently pat your skin dry with a clean, soft towel. Skin will feel soft and smooth and have a radiant glow.

STRAWBERRIES

Juicy, sweet, and reaching their peak at the height of summer, strawberries are highly alkalizing. They are packed full of fiber and vitamins—including vitamin C—and contain high levels of antioxidants, all of which helps to guard against disease and inflammation. This great-tasting and popular superfruit also aids digestion and is renowned for helping to regulate blood sugar levels.

These bright, potent fruits are rich in anthocyanins, manganese, and potassium, which help protect the heart and regulate blood pressure. Perhaps this could explain why the strawberry is considered an aphrodisiac! The combination of powerful nutrients—such as magnesium with vitamin A—helps to promote optimum skin health for a naturally radiant glow.

If you are looking for the perfect smile, look no further. Crushed strawberries mixed with a little salt provide a great natural way to whiten teeth while sweetening the breath at the same time.

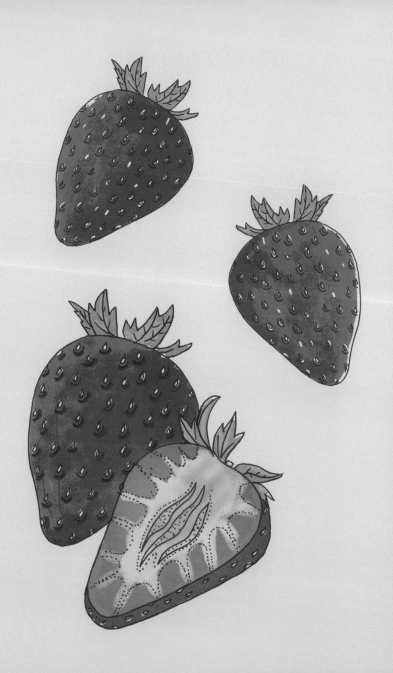

STRAWBERRY, FENNEL, AND GOAT CHEESE SALAD

Inside: Two superfoods are combined to create the perfect salad for an alkaline diet.

You will need:

2 cups strawberries • 1 large fennel bulb • 1 cucumber
• 1 small goat cheese log • 4 tablespoons olive oil
• 2 tablespoons white wine vinegar • 2 teaspoons Dijon
mustard • 1 teaspoon honey • sea salt • black pepper

To prepare:

Wash the strawberries, remove their hulls, and slice. Wash the fennel bulb, trim the fronds, remove the core, and finely slice. Wash the cucumber, then peel and finely slice. Combine the three ingredients in a large serving bowl. Cut the goat cheese into small pieces and dot over the salad.

In a separate bowl, combine the olive oil, white wine vinegar, Dijon mustard, and honey. Add sea salt and black pepper to taste. Pour the dressing over the salad and serve immediately.

GENTLE STRAWBERRY FACIAL EXFOLIATOR

Outside: Apply this enzyme-action exfoliator
for smooth and supple skin.

You will need:

1½ cups strawberries • 1 tablespoon milk • 1 tablespoon
jojoba oil

To prepare:

Mash the strawberries in a small glass bowl and mix together
with the milk and the jojoba oil.

To use:

Gently apply the exfoliant all over your cleansed face,
taking care to avoid the eyes. Leave on for five minutes (eight
minutes if you have oily skin) and rinse with warm water. Pat
dry gently, then apply your usual serum or moisturizer.

TOMATOES

Beefsteak, plum, cherry—there are several thousand varieties of this smooth-skinned superfood. Although most commonly served in salads or as a topping for Italian staples such as pasta and pizza, the tomato is actually a fruit that originated in Central America. Traditionally a summer ingredient, today the tomato tastes delicious all year round, which is great news for health and beauty.

These plump, red gems are particularly rich in lycopene, a unique and powerful antioxidant compound that helps to protect cells from free-radical damage. Lycopene is also effective in offering the skin some protection from ultraviolet (UV) rays. Tomatoes also contain high levels of potassium—a vital component of body cells and fluids—alongside calcium, iron, and manganese.

Effective levels of vitamin A and beta-carotene help to keep skin healthy and contribute to good vision, while vitamin C maintains the smooth functioning of the immune system.

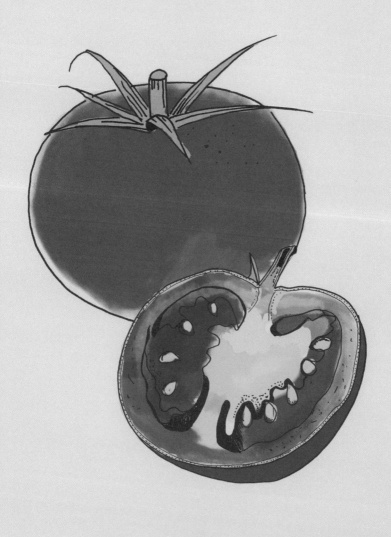

TOMATO AND BASIL BRUSCHETTA

Inside: Give your immune system a boost
with this easy lunch.

You will need:

2 teaspoons truffle oil • 2 thick-cut slices sourdough or spelt
bread • 2 ripe tomatoes • ½ avocado • pinch of dried chili flakes
• sea salt • black pepper • 2 fresh basil leaves

To prepare:

Drizzle one teaspoon of truffle oil equally across the two slices
of bread. Roughly chop the tomatoes and place in a small
bowl. Cube the avocado and add it to the bowl with the dried
chili flakes, sea salt, and black pepper to taste, and the
remaining truffle oil. Gently stir to combine and allow the
flavors to mingle.

Spoon the mixture onto the slices of bread and top each with
a fresh basil leaf, cut into strips.

TOMATO FACE MASK

Outside: Treat acne-prone or oily skin
with this deep-cleansing mask.

You will need:

2 ripe tomatoes • 1 tablespoon honey

To prepare:

Cut the tomatoes in half and scoop out the pulp and seeds into
a small bowl. Using a fork, mash the tomato flesh to a smooth
paste, add the honey, and combine thoroughly.

To use:

Smooth the paste over your face, taking care to avoid the eyes
and lips. Leave on for ten minutes, then use a washcloth to
remove. Rinse the skin with warm water and pat dry. A mild
tingling sensation is normal after applying the mask, but if it
persists or is uncomfortable, remove the mask immediately.

CHAMOMILE

Delicate German chamomile belongs to the summer-flowering daisy family and is popular as a soothing tea, best enjoyed at bedtime. Used throughout history in medicine and as a beauty treatment, this herb's calming effect can help relieve anxiety and depression, while giving the immune system a boost at the same time.

Consumed as a tea, chamomile can benefit those suffering from nausea, stomach upsets, and menstrual cramps, and can reduce colic in babies. This is because the herb increases levels of the amino acid glycine in the body, which enables muscle relaxation. A good source of antioxidants that can help regulate blood sugar, chamomile also contains traces of vitamin A and folate, as well as calcium, magnesium, and potassium.

Applied to the body, chamomile can soothe sensitive skin and help ease red patches associated with eczema, dermatitis, acne, and even sore scalps. An extra bonus for blondes: the herb can also be used as a final rinse after shampooing, lifting color for a sun-kissed effect.

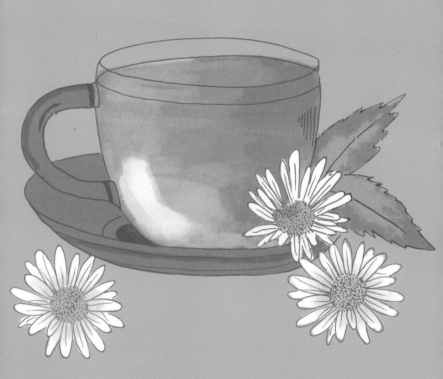

CHAMOMILE AND LEMON SPRITZ

Inside: Team calming chamomile with lemon for a refreshing alkalizer for your body.

You will need:

1 cup freshly boiled water • 5 chamomile tea bags
• 2 teaspoons raw honey • zest and juice of 1 lemon, plus a lemon slice for garnish • club soda

To prepare:

Pour the boiling water over the chamomile tea bags and leave them to infuse for five minutes to make a concentrated liquid. Remove the tea bags, then add the honey and stir to melt. Add the lemon zest and juice.

Pour the tea into a tall glass jug and add club soda to taste. Serve over ice for a refreshing and relaxing summer drink, garnished with a slice of lemon.

SLEEPY-TIME CHAMOMILE BATH SALTS

Outside: Soothe sensitive skin with this
relaxing bath time treat.

You will need:

1 cup Epsom salt • 4 chamomile tea bags or 2 tablespoons
chamomile flowers tied in a cheesecloth square

To prepare:

Place the Epsom salt and the chamomile tea bags in the
bottom of the tub and run the hot water until they are fully
covered. Allow the chamomile to infuse into the bathwater for
ten minutes, before running more water to produce the
perfect temperature for a relaxing bath.

To use:

For the maximum benefit, leave the tea bags or cloth to soak
as you relax in the bath before bedtime. This will help
promote a restful beauty sleep.

PEACHES

A delicious and aromatic stone fruit that reaches its peak at the height of summer, the peach was first cultivated in China and is now enjoyed across the globe. Sun-blushed and velvet-skinned, the juicy inner flesh of this superfruit can be yellow with a distinctive zesty flavor, or white with a sweeter tang.

Both yellow and white peaches are a great source of antioxidants, vitamins, minerals, and dietary fiber, making them an all-around superfood when promoting optimum health. Rich in immune-boosting antioxidants, including beta-carotene, which gives them their pretty orange color, peaches are especially beneficial in maintaining healthy, glowing skin. They are an excellent source of vitamin A to promote flawless skin texture and vitamin C to assist in collagen production that keeps complexions youthful. Essential minerals include potassium, magnesium, and selenium to ensure healthy cells throughout the body.

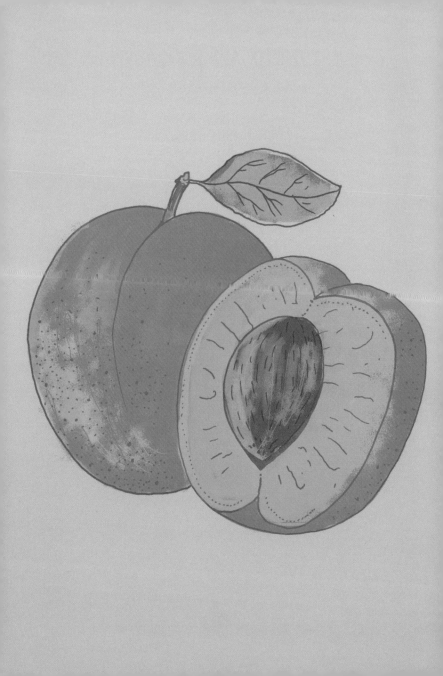

PEACH, TOMATO, AND MOZZARELLA SALAD

Inside: Invigorate skin with this antioxidant- and vitamin-rich salad.

You will need:

2 ripe peaches • 3 medium heirloom tomatoes • 1 mozzarella ball • 1 tablespoon olive oil • 1 teaspoon Dijon mustard • sea salt • black pepper • 5 basil leaves

To prepare:

Halve and pit the peaches, then cut into small chunks and place into a serving bowl. Cut the tomatoes into quarters and slice the mozzarella ball into small pieces, then add to the bowl. Mix together the olive oil, Dijon mustard, sea salt, and black pepper to taste, then pour over the ingredients in the bowl. Tear and add the basil leaves and gently combine to create a delicious healthy salad.

GENTLE PEACH EXFOLIATING MASK

Outside: Use this vitamin A–rich exfoliating mask
to encourage cell turnover.

You will need:

1 ripe peach • 1 tablespoon honey • 2 tablespoons rolled oats

To prepare:

Peel and halve the peach. Discard the pit and mash the fruit
into a purée in a small glass bowl. Add the honey and oats and
combine to form a thick paste.

To use:

Smooth the mixture over your cleansed face, avoiding the eye
area. Leave on for fifteen minutes, then massage gently to
remove loosened skin cells. Rinse your face with warm water
and pat dry with a clean, soft towel to leave glowing,
refreshed skin ready for your serum or moisturizer.

CINNAMON

Harvested from the bark of a tree native to Sri Lanka, cinnamon is a highly powerful antioxidant. Thanks to its distinctive aroma and delicious, almost sweet, flavor, this spice features in many recipes for warming baked goods and is frequently associated with winter celebrations. That's a good thing, too, since this woody superfood harbors naturally effective antimicrobial properties that make it a great support to the body's immune system during the cold and flu season.

Cinnamon is also a great source of manganese—essential for the healthy function of the metabolism and the nervous system, as well as the formation of connective tissues, maintenance of healthy bones, and the regulation of blood sugar levels. Mixing a teaspoon of cinnamon with raw honey can help soothe sore throats or ease respiratory problems, while some find the scent of cinnamon helps boost concentration and brain activity!

The health and beauty benefits of this superspice can be enjoyed throughout the year by adding a light sprinkling to cereal and yogurt or as a finishing touch to a cup of coffee or hot chocolate.

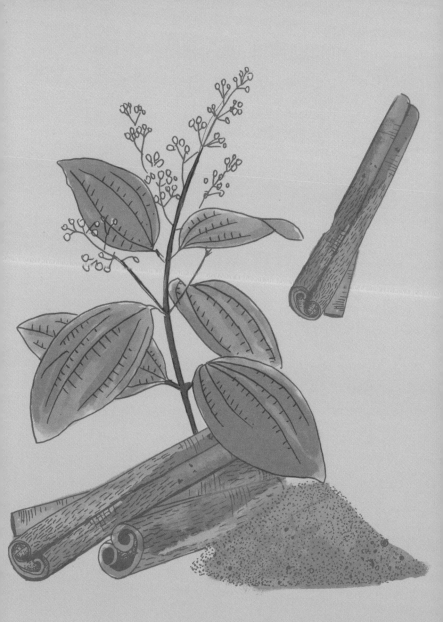

CINNAMON AND GINGER MELON

Inside: Enjoy the calming effects of this
refreshing and fruity concoction.

You will need:

½ cantaloupe • ½ honeydew • ½-inch piece fresh ginger • 1 cup
water • 1 cinnamon stick • 1 teaspoon ground cinnamon
• ¾ cup coconut sugar • juice of ½ lemon • Greek yogurt

To prepare:

Cut the melons into equal-sized cubes and place in a serving
bowl. Peel and finely chop the ginger and place in a small
saucepan with the water, cinnamon stick, ground cinnamon,
coconut sugar, and lemon juice.

Heat over medium heat until the sugar has melted, then
simmer over low heat until the mixture has reduced and
thickened to a light syrup. Pour over the melon cubes and
decorate with the cinnamon stick. Serve with a dollop of
Greek yogurt.

CINNAMON SPOT TREATMENT

Outside: Reduce the redness of acne with this deep-clean treatment.

You will need:

1 tablespoon honey • ½ teaspoon ground cinnamon

To prepare:

Combine the honey and cinnamon together to form a thick, smooth paste.

To use:

Use a cotton swab to dab a generous amount of the paste onto the affected area(s). Leave for ten minutes then rinse away. Repeat morning and evening.

MANGOES

Delicious, nutritious, and the ultimate symbol of summer, the mango is a real feel-good fruit. Commended for aiding concentration, weight loss, and digestion, it also restores elasticity and hydration for youthful-looking skin and healthy hair. Mangoes are packed with vitamins and minerals that regulate, cleanse, and nourish the body. They contain high levels of probiotic fiber, making this smooth-skinned superfruit a healthy, belly-friendly snack or dessert.

The mango's high levels of alkaline-balancing tartaric and malic acids, as well as powerful vitamins A and C, help boost the immune system and keep eyes clear and healthy. B vitamins are great for balancing hormones and keeping the heart healthy, while rich sources of iron, calcium, beta-carotene, potassium, magnesium, and copper help keep blood, skin, and hair in tip-top condition.

Although naturally sweet when ripe, mangoes have a low glycemic index (41–60) so you won't experience the kind of "sugar rush" you have after eating a chocolate bar. Nevertheless, you will feel full, satisfied, and blessed with healthy energy.

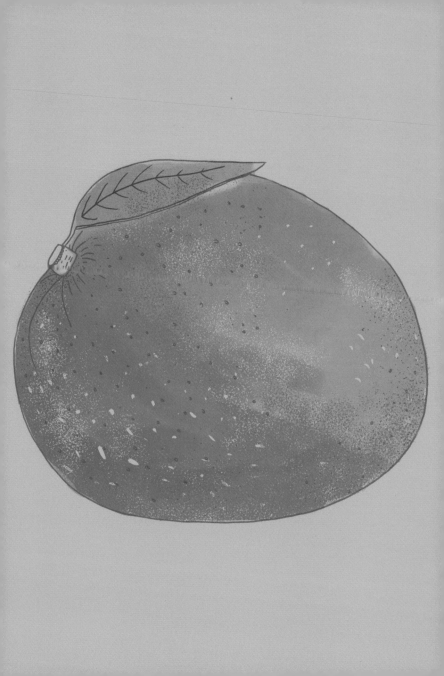

MANGO SALSA

Inside: Eat this fiery, probiotic salsa to aid digestion.

You will need:

2 ripe mangoes • 1 small red onion • 1 small red chili • 1 tablespoon extra-virgin olive oil • juice of ½ lime • ½ bunch fresh cilantro leaves • sea salt • black pepper

To prepare:

Peel and pit the mangoes and slice into strips. Finely chop the red onion and the chili, taking care to remove the chili seeds. Place all together in a small serving bowl and add the olive oil and the lime juice.

Top with torn cilantro leaves and mix to combine, adding sea salt and black pepper to taste. Cover and refrigerate for thirty minutes to allow the flavors to combine before serving.

MANGO AND AVOCADO CLEANSER

Outside: Enrich your skin with this nourishing
cocktail of vitamins and good oils.

You will need:

1 ripe mango • ½ ripe avocado • 1 tablespoon yogurt

To prepare:

Place the flesh of the mango and the avocado in a small dish
and add the yogurt. Mash, then mix to a smooth consistency.

To use:

Gently massage the cleanser onto your face, neck, and
décolletage for around three minutes. Rinse with warm water
and pat dry before applying your usual serum or moisturizer.
For a deeper cleanse, keep the face mask on for ten minutes
before rinsing.

PAPAYAS

At its best in early summer, a ripe papaya is delicious simply with a squeeze of lime. It also combines well with other fruits or vegetables to make a delicious low-calorie smoothie or dessert.

Green, or unripe, papaya is popular in savory, Asian style dishes and contains high levels of papain, an enzyme that naturally tenderizes meat. This tropical superfruit also contains high amounts of phytonutrients, minerals, and vitamins, as well as soluble dietary fiber, which aids digestion. With a higher vitamin C content than even a lemon, the papaya is a great immune booster.

Potent levels of vitamin A, beta-carotene, and lutein combine with essential B-complex vitamins, potassium, and calcium to make the papaya a powerful antioxidant that will keep you in the very best of health—from your hair right down to your toenails.

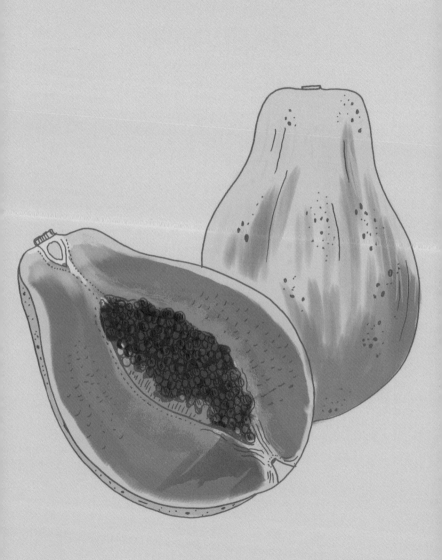

PAPAYA, AVOCADO, AND CUCUMBER SALAD

Inside: Combine this trio of superfoods for glossy hair and glowing skin.

You will need:

1 ripe papaya • 1 ripe avocado • ½ cucumber • ½ bunch fresh mint • 1 tablespoon olive oil • juice of ½ lemon • sea salt • black pepper

To prepare:

Peel the papaya, remove the seeds, and cut the flesh into slices. Repeat with the avocado and place both in a serving bowl. Cut the cucumber into chunks, add to the bowl and top with torn, fresh mint leaves. Prepare the dressing by mixing the olive oil and lemon juice with sea salt and black pepper to taste.

Pour the dressing over the salad and toss gently before serving. This salad pairs well with roasted chicken.

HONEY AND PAPAYA TREATMENT FOR HANDS AND FEET

Outside: Smooth rough or dry skin with
this enzyme-rich mix.

You will need:

½ ripe papaya • 3 tablespoons honey • 1 tablespoon
rolled oats

To prepare:

Scoop out the flesh of the papaya into a small glass bowl,
mash, and add the honey and the oats. Combine thoroughly.

To use:

Soak your hands and feet in warm water for five minutes,
pat dry, then coat with the papaya mixture. Leave for thirty
minutes before massaging the mixture gently into your skin.
Rinse in warm water to remove.

SWEET POTATOES

Native to Central and South America, the sweet potato was introduced to Europe by Christopher Columbus toward the end of the fifteenth century. It was not long before its popularity spread across the rest of the globe. Although most of us see orange when we think of this starchy tuber, purple varieties grow, too.

Orange or purple, this supertuber is rich in manganese, copper, essential B vitamins, potassium, phosphorus, and fiber. It also contains choline—a nutrient that helps maintain cell membranes and the transmission of cell impulses. Consequently, it assists with muscle movement, memory, and sleep. Sweet potatoes are high in the phytonutrient beta-carotene, which the body converts to vitamin A, and in anti-inflammatory anthocyanins. Combined with slow-release carbohydrates, this is all good news for blood-sugar regulation.

Cook this root vegetable in its skin with a small amount of fat. That way you'll get the maximum benefits from all it has to offer.

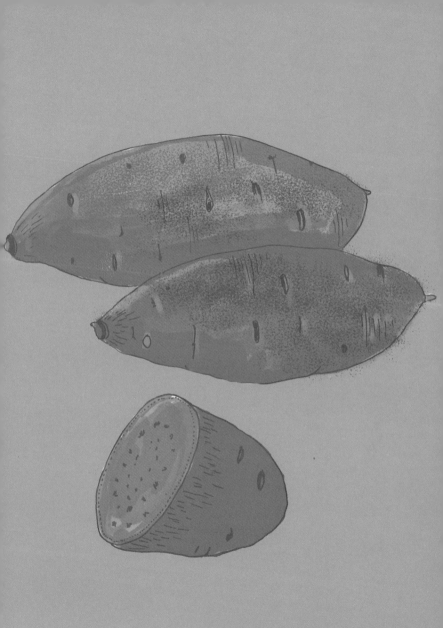

SCRUMPTIOUS SWEET POTATO SMASH

Inside: Top up your beta-carotene levels for a boost
of anti-inflammatory vitamin A.

You will need:

2 sweet potatoes • 1 tablespoon ghee or olive oil • 2 tablespoons
grated Parmesan • sea salt • black pepper

To prepare:

Scrub the sweet potatoes and cut them into small cubes,
leaving the peel on. Place in a medium saucepan, cover with
water, and boil until the flesh is soft, then strain. Add the
ghee or olive oil and mash the cubes lightly with a fork. Add
sea salt and black pepper to taste.

Transfer the mashed potatoes to an ovenproof serving dish,
top with the grated Parmesan, and broil until golden brown.
Serve immediately with fish or chicken.

SWEET POTATO
DÉCOLLETAGE RUB

Outside: Exfoliate and moisturize with this
hydrating skin treatment.

You will need:

1 sweet potato • 1 tablespoon yogurt • 1 tablespoon coconut oil

To prepare:

Peel and cube the sweet potato and boil until soft. Add the
yogurt and coconut oil and combine thoroughly to make a
paste, using a hand blender for a smoother result, if desired.

To use:

Smooth the paste over your décolletage and neck. Leave for
fifteen minutes to exfoliate, hydrate, and nourish this delicate
area. You can also use this treatment all over your face, taking
care to avoid the eye area.

ALMONDS

Nutrient dense and with a high (good) fat content,
a handful of almonds makes the perfect beauty snack.

An excellent source of vitamin E, B vitamins, potassium, calcium,
magnesium, phosphorus, and iron, as well as essential mono- and
polyunsaturated fatty acids, the almond is a powerhouse of goodness
that will literally make skin and hair glow and encourage strong nails.
These sweet, milky kernels are also rich in antioxidants, which help
keep the whole body healthy—even the heart.

Enjoy almonds raw or dry roasted—or soak them overnight before
adding to breakfast cereal (this makes the nutrients more easily
digestible). A truly versatile superfood, the almond's benefits can also
be found in a glass of almond milk, in almond butter, or in
cookies made with almond meal.

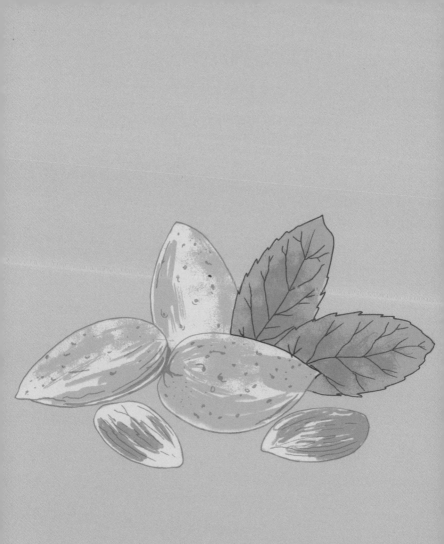

ALMOND BREAKFAST SMOOTHIE

Inside: Give your skin a healthy glow with this magnesium- and vitamin E-rich smoothie.

You will need:

1 cup almond milk • 1 banana • 1 cup frozen raspberries
• 1 tablespoon almond butter • 1 teaspoon honey • 1 tablespoon rolled oats (optional) • ground cinnamon

To prepare:

Place all the ingredients except the cinnamon in a blender and blitz together to make a thick and creamy smoothie. Dust the top with cinnamon and serve immediately.

SWEET ALMOND OIL FACIAL CLEANSER

Outside: Apply this nutty treatment for smooth, supple, and hydrated skin.

You will need:

4 tablespoons sweet almond oil • 2 tablespoons coconut oil • small glass jar with a screw-top lid

To prepare:

Pour the two oils into the glass jar, screw on the lid, and shake to combine thoroughly. Store in the refrigerator.

To use:

Gently warm the oil between your fingertips before massaging all over your face to loosen makeup and grime. Rinse a washcloth in warm water and then gently wipe across your face to remove the cleansing oil and surface grime. Rinse the cloth thoroughly and leave to air dry.

CIDER VINEGAR

Cider vinegar has been credited with amazing health benefits for centuries. It is made by crushing apples and then adding yeast to ferment the natural sugars. A bacteria is introduced, which turns the liquid into acetic acid. Small quantities of proteins, enzymes, and healthy bacteria then form, which are believed to give this tangy superfood its antioxidant, antibacterial, and antimicrobial qualities.

A great balancing act, cider vinegar is helpful in restoring healthy bacteria in the stomach, resulting in better digestion and higher energy levels. At the same time, it can help regulate blood sugar and cholesterol levels. Mixed with honey and lemon juice, cider vinegar is a useful antioxidant-rich treatment for colds during winter months, killing bacteria and soothing sore throats. Used externally, it is an ideal all-natural cleaning fluid!

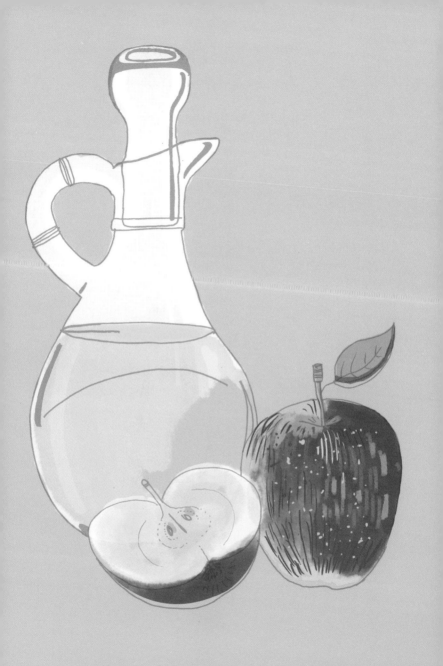

CIDER VINEGAR MARY

Inside: Mix up this taste bud–tingling
tomato juice to ease digestion.

You will need:

1 cup fresh tomato juice • 2 tablespoons cider vinegar
• 1 splash Worcestershire sauce • sea salt • black pepper
• celery stick

To prepare:

Pour the tomato juice into a tall glass and add the cider
vinegar and Worcestershire sauce. Sprinkle with sea salt and
black pepper to taste. Stir with the celery stick before serving.

SUPER SCALP CLEANSER

Outside: Soothe a flaky scalp with this naturally
antimicrobial, enzyme-action rinse.

You will need:

1 cup cider vinegar • 1 cup water • 2 drops lavender oil

To prepare:

Mix the cider vinegar and the water together, then add the
lavender oil and stir.

To use:

To treat an itchy, flaky scalp, gently massage the mixture into
your scalp. Leave for twenty minutes to allow the cider
vinegar to alter the pH balance, then rinse, and shampoo and
condition as usual. For the ultimate shine treatment, use the
mixture in the final rinse after washing your hair.

HONEY

A product of the bee's hard labor, honey plays a vital role in the ecology of the planet. It also happens to be a golden elixir that has been used for centuries as a delicious superfood and a highly effective medicine. Powerful antioxidant, antibacterial, and antimicrobial benefits bring an impressive boost to the immune system while protecting against aging and infection—even when applied topically.

With high levels of fructose and glucose, both of which are easily absorbed by the body, honey gives an instant energy boost. B-complex vitamins are also present, alongside calcium, copper, iron, magnesium, manganese, phosphorus, potassium, sodium, and zinc. Important amino acids help maintain and repair the body's connective tissues.

Depending on the climate and environment of the bees, some types of honey have more powerful effects than others. For example, manuka honey is made by bees that flock to the manuka bush in New Zealand, and has particularly effective antimicrobial properties.

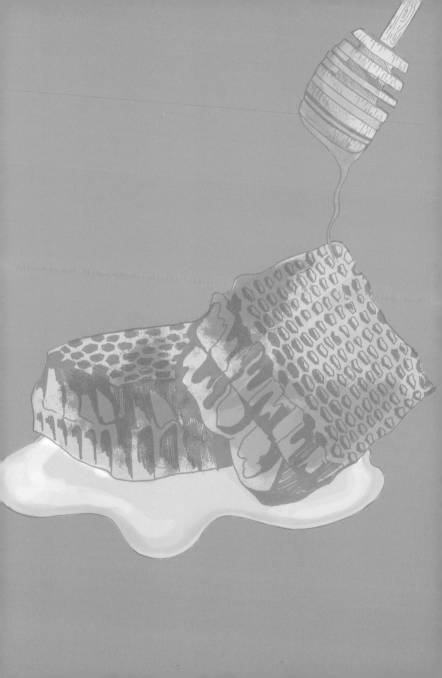

RAW SALAD WITH HONEY

Inside: Give your immune system a boost with this nutrient-rich, honey-flavored dressing.

You will need:

¼ white cabbage • 1 carrot • 1 green apple • 1 tablespoon cider vinegar • 1 tablespoon olive oil • 2 teaspoons honey • juice of ¼ lemon • chili flakes • sea salt • black pepper

To prepare:

Finely shred the white cabbage and place in a serving dish. Scrub the carrot, wash the apple, and cut both into fine julienned sticks. Add to the dish.

Pour the cider vinegar, olive oil, honey, and lemon juice into a small glass bowl and add the chili flakes. Whisk together until thoroughly combined. Add sea salt and black pepper to taste, before pouring the dressing over the serving dish. Stir well to coat the ingredients fully.

HONEY AND PEPPERMINT LIP BALM

Outside: Keep your lips hydrated in winter with this antibacterial lip treatment.

You will need:

1 tablespoon coconut oil • 1 teaspoon honey • 2 drops peppermint oil • small glass jar with screw-top lid

To prepare:

Spoon the coconut oil and honey into a small glass bowl. Place the bowl over a small saucepan of boiling water and heat until thoroughly melted and combined. Remove from the heat.

Once the mixture has cooled, add the peppermint oil and stir thoroughly. Pour into the jar. Allow to cool and firm up before screwing on the lid.

To use:

Apply the tingly lip balm to your lips for soothing hydration.

LEMONS

With their powerful immune-boosting, antioxidant, antibacterial, and antiviral properties, lemons have amazing natural healing properties that offer great health and beauty benefits, inside and out. Although lemons taste acidic, they are actually alkaline, which means they help to regulate the body to an ideal balance of pH 7.30–7.45. Lemon juice also aids digestion and helps cleanse the liver. This all adds up to a healthier body, which means clearer skin and shinier hair!

But it doesn't stop there. The mighty lemon offers 88 percent of your daily dose of vitamin C—renowned for fighting colds and flu bugs—along with potassium and magnesium, both of which help promote healthy skin. For double the impact, lemons can be used in a number of beauty treatments to cleanse, refresh, and add a youthful glow: skin looks more radiant, hair looks shinier, and nails look whiter with a little help from the humble lemon. One easy way to include lemon in your daily routine is to squeeze the juice of half a lemon into a glass of room-temperature water, then sip first thing in the morning.

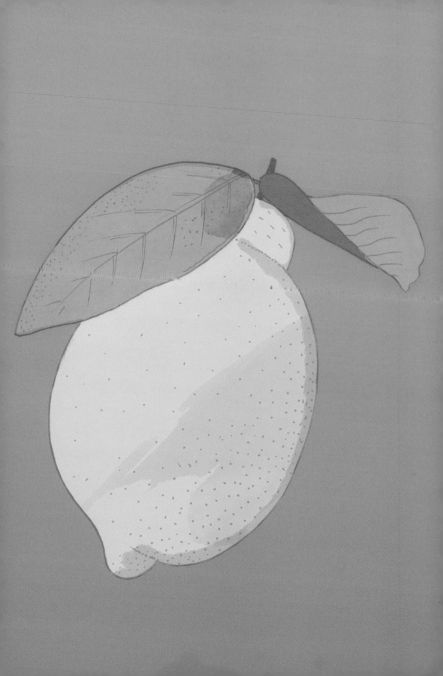

LEMON AND PARSLEY LENTIL SALAD

Inside: Eat this refreshing, alkalizing, and cleansing salad for an all-over body glow.

You will need:

1 red pepper • 1 cucumber • 1 small red onion • 2½ cups cooked brown lentils • small bunch fresh parsley • juice of 1 lemon • 2 teaspoons Dijon mustard • ¼ teaspoon sea salt • black pepper • ⅓ cup extra-virgin olive oil

To prepare:

Chop the red pepper, the cucumber, and the red onion and place in a large bowl. Add the cooked lentils. Chop the parsley and place in a blender with the lemon juice, mustard, sea salt, and black pepper, then gradually add the olive oil to emulsify and create the dressing.

Pour the dressing into the bowl and mix all the ingredients together. Serve with a broiled chicken breast or poached fish.

LEMON AND HONEY FACE MASK

Outside: Revive dry skin with this exfoliating, soothing, and moisturizing treatment.

You will need:

4 tablespoons lemon juice • 4 tablespoons honey

• 4 tablespoons almond oil

To prepare:

Mix together the lemon juice, honey, and almond oil in a small bowl.

To use:

Apply the mask to your face, taking care to avoid the eye area. Leave for fifteen minutes, then rinse off with warm water and pat dry. Your skin will feel soft, smooth, and moisturized. To help brighten areas of skin pigmentation or acne scars, add an extra tablespoon of lemon juice and reduce the quantity of almond oil.

OATS

Traditionally a favorite winter breakfast, oats are a supergrain containing important nutrients that help maintain a healthy body and glowing skin. They are a great source of both soluble and nonsoluble dietary fiber. Beta-glucan is a soluble fiber in oats that can lower cholesterol and regulate blood sugar levels, while the nonsoluble fiber in oats helps to keep the digestive system healthy.

Phytoestrogen helps to keep hormones balanced, while a high carbohydrate and protein content, along with essential fatty acids, important B complex vitamins, and vitamin E, contribute to optimum health and energy.

Oats also contain a good level of calcium, manganese, zinc, selenium, copper, iron, and magnesium—essential for the smooth functioning and repair of the body, including skin, hair, and nails—making them an all-around great beauty superfood.

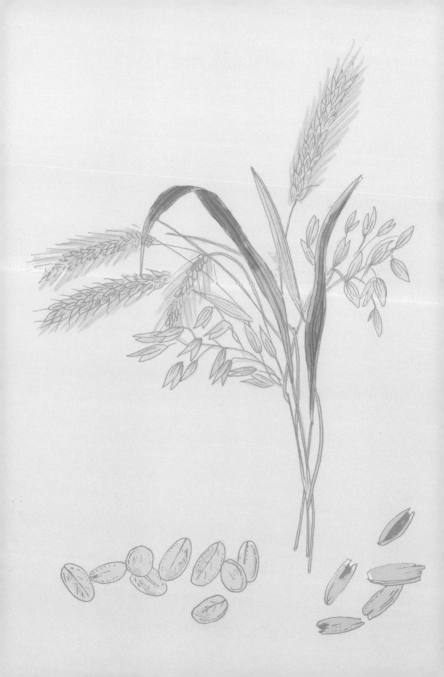

BIRCHER MUESLI

Inside: Calm your digestive system
with this oaty breakfast.

You will need:

1 cup rolled oats • 1 apple • 2 pitted dates • 1 tablespoon
roasted chopped hazelnuts • 1 tablespoon dried goji berries
• 2–3 tablespoons yogurt

To prepare:

Place the oats in a bowl, add just enough water to cover, and
soak overnight. Grate the apple, chop the dates, and add to the
soaked oats along with the chopped hazelnuts and goji berries.
Add enough yogurt to bind all the ingredients, plus a little
more to taste.

OAT AND LAVENDER BATH SOAK

Outside: Restore health to your skin with
this soothing bath time treat.

You will need:

½ cup rolled oats • 2 tablespoons milk powder • 4 drops
lavender oil • cheesecloth square • string

To prepare:

In a small bowl, combine the rolled oats with the milk powder
and add the lavender oil. Spoon into the center of the
cheesecloth, then gather the edges and tie with the string.

To use:

Place the bag in a running bathtub and leave to soak, like a tea
bag, as you bathe. It will leave your skin feeling soothed and
smooth. You will also feel relaxed and ready to enjoy a good
night's sleep.

PINEAPPLES

A potent symbol of tropical goodness, the pineapple is fresh tasting and packed with low-calorie goodness. Its zesty sharpness comes from the presence of the enzyme bromelain, which helps maintain a healthy digestive system by breaking down protein in food. Consequently, the pineapple is a great natural detox food and, thanks to a high fiber content, it is also beneficial for weight loss.

An excellent source of vitamin C and other cell-protecting antioxidants, pineapples not only aid in collagen production for healthy skin, but also provide a helpful surge to the immune system, making them a great choice in winter.

Pineapple is known for its high level of manganese— a mineral that is essential in energy production—and thiamine, which promotes healthy bones. Copper and potassium assist with the production of red blood cells, contributing to healthy heart function.

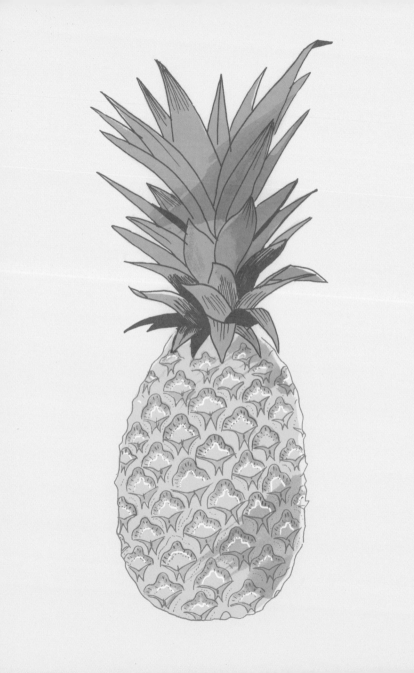

TROPICAL PINEAPPLE AND COCONUT

Inside: Increase your fiber intake with this
seemingly decadent dessert.

You will need:

$^1/_3$ pineapple • ¼ cup muscovado sugar • ½ cup coconut milk
• mint leaves

To prepare:

Peel the pineapple and cut into thick rings, then quarter the
rings. Place on a baking sheet and sprinkle with muscovado
sugar. Broil for three to five minutes, until brown. Remove
from the broiler and serve drizzled with coconut milk and
garnished with mint leaves.

PINEAPPLE FOOT SCRUB

Outside: Smooth feet and polish toenails
with this enzyme-acting scrub.

You will need:

2 tablespoons coconut oil • 2 cups fresh pineapple chunks

• plastic wrap • foot file

To prepare:

Gently heat the coconut oil and blend or mash together with
the pineapple chunks to make a mask.

To use:

Smooth the mask onto the soles of your feet and cover with
plastic wrap to form socks. Leave for fifteen minutes to allow
the pineapple's enzymes to soften any hard skin. Meanwhile,
the coconut oil will condition your feet. Remove the plastic
wrap, rinse your feet in warm water, and gently file to remove
dead skin. Your feet will feel baby soft and smooth!

AVOCADOS

Healthy fats are important for the body to function at its best and eating half an avocado will provide 18g of very beneficial monounsaturated fat. In addition to helping disperse fat-soluble vitamins E and K around the body, monounsaturated fat is vital for maintaining the moisture levels in skin that keep it feeling soft and looking evenly toned and healthy. Hair feels softer and more silky and nails are more resilient. Vitamin E in avocados helps protect skin from visible signs of aging, while vitamin C assists in the creation of elastin and collagen to keep skin looking youthful.

Avocados contain folate and potassium, vital for maintaining the nervous system and a healthy heart. Like all superfoods, they offer valuable anti-inflammatory and antioxidant protection. Simply adding a little of this superfruit to your salad or to a daily smoothie can make a world of difference to your general health and appearance. Enjoy a long season of this king of fruits from spring to fall.

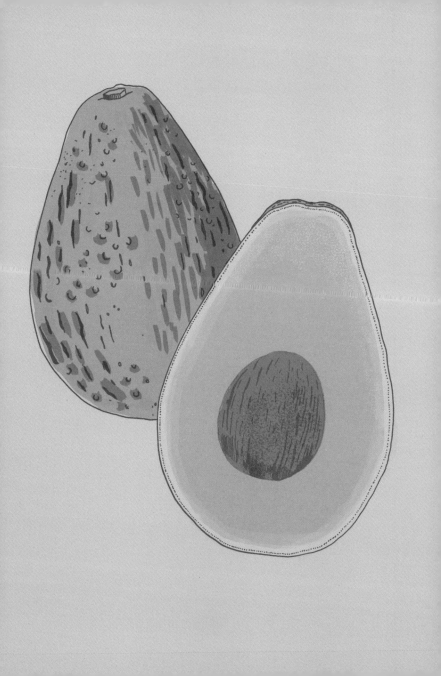

GREEN BREAKFAST SMOOTHIE

Inside: Drink this rich-tasting smoothie to give your body an alkaline boost.

You will need:

½ ripe avocado • 1 ripe banana • 1 kiwifruit • 1 handful chopped kale • 1 cup milk (dairy, soy, or rice) • ¼ teaspoon cinnamon • 1 teaspoon honey

To prepare:

Place all the ingredients in a blender and blend until smooth. Pour into a glass and serve immediately.

AVOCADO HAIR TREATMENT

Outside: Bring your split ends under control
with this tropical-smelling blend.

You will need:

2 tablespoons coconut oil • ½ avocado

To prepare:

Melt one tablespoon of the coconut oil in a small bowl placed
over a small saucepan of boiling water. Remove the bowl from
the double boiler and add the avocado flesh, mashing to combine
until very smooth.

To use:

Before shampooing your hair, warm the remaining coconut oil
until clear and gently massage it into your scalp and roots. Comb
the avocado mixture through to the ends of your hair. Leave on
for ten minutes, then rinse with warm water before shampooing
as normal.

Try this treatment once a month to hydrate and condition hair.

COCONUTS

This tropical superfruit is loaded with vitamins—predominantly C and B—plus minerals and is high in antioxidant, antiaging compounds with anti-inflammatory, antibacterial, and antiviral benefits for all areas of the body. When young, coconuts have an outer green husk and softer, more creamy "meat." As coconuts mature, they develop a brown husk and the meat is much firmer. Green coconut "meat" is rich in calcium and important fatty acids, while coconut oil has great antioxidant power that is retained even when heated during cooking.

Although green and mature coconuts both contain coconut water, the level of beneficial nutrients is much higher in the green coconut. With good levels of iron, calcium, manganese, magnesium, copper, and phosphorus, and impressively rich in potassium, green coconut water is ideal for restoring electrolyte levels during hot weather. It is also supremely hydrating, which is great news for skin and muscles. The water also makes an effective treatment for stomach upsets and can help regulate blood sugar levels.

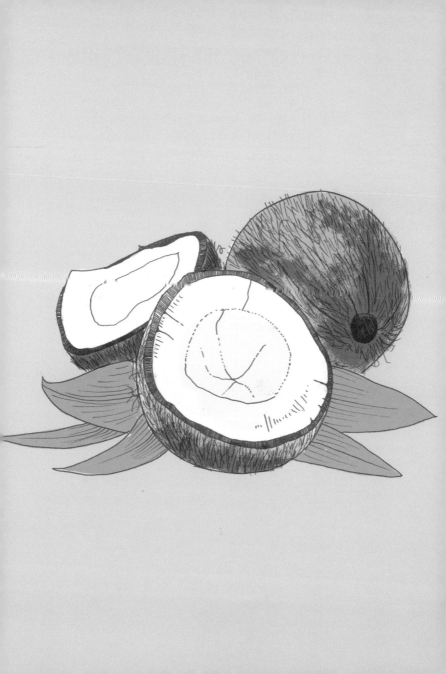

GREEN COCONUT AND MANGO CREAM

Inside: Give your immune system a boost with this delicious treat, rich in vitamins A and C.

You will need:

1 green coconut • 1 ripe mango • 1 teaspoon honey (optional)

To prepare:

Remove the top of the green coconut using a sharp knife. Pour out the coconut water and set aside. Use a spoon to scoop out the green coconut meat and place in a blender. Slice the mango on either side of the pit and scoop out the flesh. Add to the coconut in the blender and blend thoroughly, adding a little of the coconut water, until the mixture forms a rich cream. Add the honey to taste.

Serve the cream as a topping for blueberries, strawberries, or raspberries, or enjoy on its own with toasted, sliced almonds.

COCONUT OIL AND LAVENDER BODY CREAM

Outside: Nourish all skin, even sensitive types, with this super-hydrating ointment.

You will need:

1 cup coconut oil • 4 drops lavender oil • small glass jar with screw-top lid

To prepare:

Spoon the coconut oil into a glass bowl and place over a small saucepan of boiling water until melted. Add the lavender oil and combine thoroughly, then remove from the heat.

Allow to cool and firm up, until almost solid. Then, using a hand blender or a whisk, beat the mixture until it becomes light and creamy. Spoon into the jar and seal, until ready to use.

To use:

Smooth the mixture over dry skin to moisturize and help you relax before bedtime.

CUCUMBERS

A popular ingredient in summer salads, cucumbers are rich in
nutrients and contain two of the essential elements for healthy
digestion: water and fiber. Approximately 96 percent water, this
refreshing superfood is a great cleanser, helping to flush out toxins
that can dull the skin and hair. High levels of the minerals magnesium,
potassium, and silicon help restore a healthy, youthful glow to the
skin and bring a glossy sheen to the hair. Vitamins A and C provide
an immune boost that results in a natural radiance, while vitamin K
ensures healthy capillaries and a strong nervous system.

Cucumbers can also have a calming effect: significant levels of vitamins
B1, B5, and B7 are important for relieving anxiety and the effects of
stress, while potassium helps reduce blood pressure and protects the
heart. So there is some truth to the phrase "cool as a cucumber," both
inside and out, as it happens, since everyone knows that a slice of
cucumber is a great way to cool and soothe a sore eye.

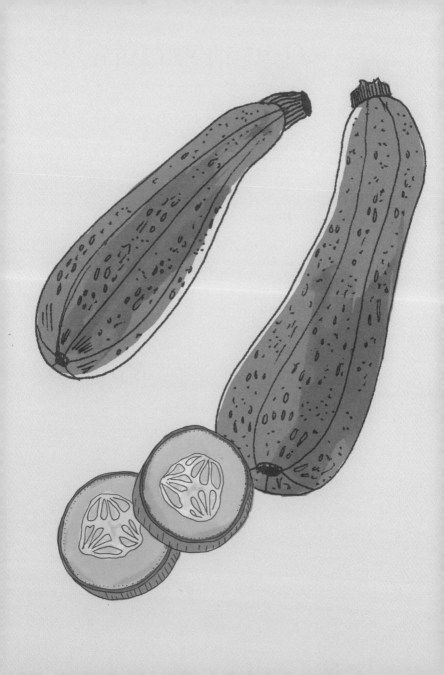

CUCUMBER AND MINT RAITA

Inside: Eat this cleansing side dish for glowing skin and shiny hair.

You will need:

1 cup yogurt • 1 tablespoon freshly chopped mint
• juice of ½ lime • 1 teaspoon cumin • 1 cucumber • sea salt
• black pepper

To prepare:

Stir the yogurt, mint, lime juice, and cumin together in a small glass bowl. Finely chop the cucumber, leaving the skin on, and add to the yogurt mix, seasoning with sea salt and black pepper to taste. The raita is delicious served as a salad dressing or as a perfect accompaniment to curries or spicy food.

COOLING FACE AND BODY MIST

Outside: Hydrate both face and body with this refreshing, mineral-rich mist.

You will need:

2 cucumbers • ½ cup rose water • cheesecloth square

• 8 oz spray bottle

To prepare:

Wash the cucumbers and finely grate them into a glass bowl. Squeeze through the cheesecloth into a second glass bowl to extract the cucumber water. Combine with the rose water, then pour into the spray bottle.

To use:

Spray over the face and body to condition and cool throughout the hot summer months. Stored in the refrigerator, this mist will last for seven days.

FENNEL

With their delicate aniseed flavor, fennel bulbs are popular in
salads and as a cooked vegetable in Mediterranean cuisine. Harvested
during the winter months, fennel has many health benefits, including
soothing digestive problems, helping your body get the maximum
health and beauty benefits from the superfoods you eat.

Fennel contains folic acid, which is essential for healthy cell
development. It also has significant levels of vitamin C—important for
a healthy immune system, as well as potassium for regulating blood
pressure and keeping cells and fluids at their optimum functionality.
Small quantities of trace minerals iron, calcium, magnesium,
manganese, zinc, copper, and selenium help to bring out
the best in skin, hair, and nails.

Finally, fennel's essential oil is often used in toothpaste and
mouthwash for its antibacterial and antifungal properties.

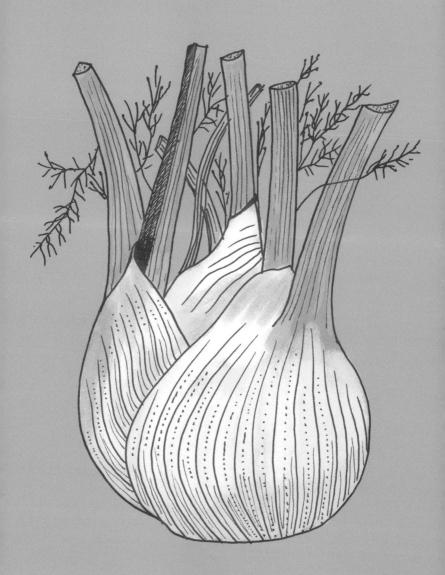

FENNEL, ORANGE, AND MINT SALAD

Inside: Give your skin, hair, and nails a welcome
boost with this mineral-rich salad.

You will need:

1 bulb fennel • 1 navel orange • 1 tablespoon olive oil • juice of
¼ lemon • sea salt • black pepper • ½ bunch fresh mint

To prepare:

Trim the fennel bulb, cut into wafer-thin slices, and arrange
on a serving plate. Using a sharp knife, peel the orange and
cut into segments, removing the pith. Arrange the orange
segments over the fennel slices and squeeze over any
additional orange juice.

Mix the olive oil and lemon juice together and add sea salt and
black pepper to taste. Pour the dressing over the salad. Chop
the mint leaves and sprinkle over the salad before serving.

FENNEL SEED EYE COMFORT

Outside: Reduce puffiness or redness to leave
your eyes looking clear and bright.

You will need:

1 cup water • 2 teaspoons fennel seeds • small glass jar with
screw-top lid

To prepare:

Boil the water and pour over the fennel seeds in the glass jar.
Leave to infuse for five minutes, before straining the seeds
and allowing the eyewash to cool. Store in the refrigerator.

To use:

Soak two cotton balls in the fennel eyewash and place over
closed eyes for ten minutes.

GREEN TEA

Recognized as one of the healthiest drinks available, green tea
contains a range of important nutrients to ensure a healthy
mind, body, and soul!

This refreshing elixir is rich in polyphenols, which have a powerful
antioxidant and anti-inflammatory effect on the body, protecting
cells and molecules from free-radical damage. The drink also contains
small quantities of amino acids and minerals that help keep the body
functioning well and can even help lower cholesterol levels
and maintain a healthy metabolic rate.

Flavonoids called catechins can help to slow down bacteria and virus
growth, making green tea a great choice in wintertime. Surprisingly,
for a healthy drink, this superfood also contains caffeine. Often
considered a negative property in a drink, caffeine is, in fact, an
important stimulant for the brain, promoting improved concentration,
memory, reaction time, and even mood. However, as with all food and
drink, the advice is not to overdo it!

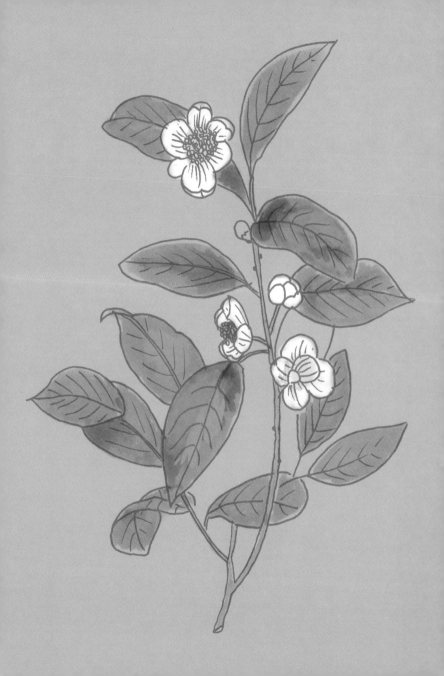

GREEN TEA WITH MINT AND GINGER

Inside: Drink this winter warmer
to soothe a sore throat.

You will need:

1 green tea bag • 4 fresh mint leaves • small piece
fresh ginger • 1 cup freshly boiled water

To prepare:

Place the tea bag, mint leaves, and a little grated ginger in a
cup. Pour freshly boiled water into the cup and allow the
ingredients to infuse for three minutes. Remove the tea bag
and mint leaves before drinking.

GREEN TEA
STEAM FACIAL TREATMENT

Outside: Combine green tea and lavender for
a powerful antibacterial cleanser.

You will need:

2 green tea bags • 1 cup freshly boiled water • 4 drops lavender oil

To prepare:

Place the tea bags in a small bowl and cover with freshly
boiled water. Allow to infuse for two minutes—it should be
cooler but still steaming—then add the lavender oil.

To use:

Lean your face over the bowl with a hand-width distance
from your nose to the water. Breathe deeply, allowing the
steam to open your pores. Stay in this position as long as is
comfortable, then gently splash cool water over your face
to refresh and close the pores.

MINT

Fresh mint is a popular herb used all over the world for adding a zesty, refreshing flavor to a dish, as a garnish, and as a tea. Although there are around fifteen to twenty different types of mint, the most commonly used are spearmint and peppermint. Both grow all year round indoors and thrive outdoors in the summer sunshine.

Mint not only tastes great, it contains small amounts of vitamins A and C, potassium, calcium, phosphorus, magnesium, and iron—all important nutrients for healthy skin. It also contains menthol, which works as a decongestant. However, the herb's greatest benefit is the potent antioxidant power it derives from rosmarinic acid, which has proved effective in relieving inflammation and treating a number of other allergy symptoms.

Mint is great to drink as a tea when you have a cold. It relieves sore throats and congestion. It also relieves indigestion and irritable bowel syndrome. When applied to the skin, mint cools and calms redness associated with common skin rashes or insect bites.

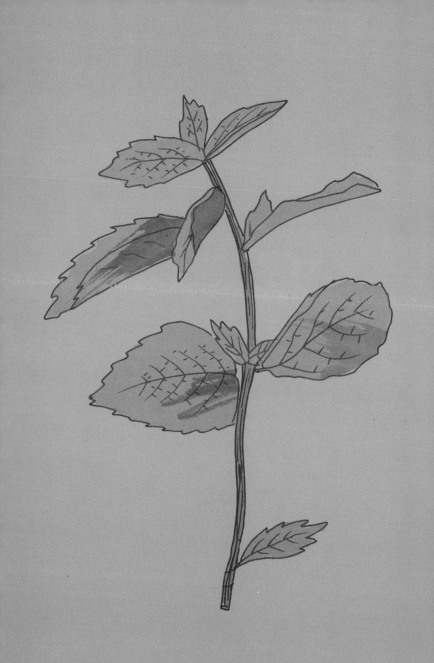

ZINGY MINTY SALAD

Inside: Enjoy this clean-tasting salad for
an antioxidant boost.

You will need:

¼ watermelon • 1 cucumber • 7 oz feta cheese • 1 bunch
fresh mint leaves • juice of 1 lime • sea salt • black pepper

To prepare:

Chop the watermelon into dice-sized cubes, remove any seeds,
and place in a serving bowl. Trim and peel the cucumber and
slice into thin rounds. Dice the feta and tear or chop the mint
leaves, reserving a few whole leaves for garnish. Add the
cucumber, feta, and mint to the serving bowl. Pour the lime
juice over the fruit and sprinkle with a pinch of sea salt and
black pepper to taste.

Gently mix all the ingredients to combine thoroughly, then
top with the reserved mint leaves. Serve chilled.

REFRESHING MINT HAIR RINSE

Outside: Refresh and soothe your scalp
while adding extra gloss to your hair.

You will need:

1 peppermint tea bag • 1 teaspoon dried lavender or
chamomile flowers • ½ cup freshly boiled water
• 2 tablespoons cider vinegar

To prepare:

Place the tea bag and the dried lavender or chamomile flowers
in a small bowl and cover with the freshly boiled water.
Strain to remove the tea bag and dried flowers, then stir in the
cider vinegar.

To use:

Shampoo and condition your hair as usual. Then, for the final
rinse, gently massage your scalp and hair with the minty
solution. Dry and style your hair as usual.

BLACK GRAPES

Available all year round, rich, blue-black grapes feature regularly in a healthy Mediterranean diet and are filled with highly beneficial phytonutrients. Their dark color comes from anthocyanins— anti-inflammatory antioxidant compounds that boost the immune system and keep the skin and body in the best of health

Black grapes also contain another highly powerful antioxidant, resveratrol, which helps to maintain a healthy circulatory system, ensuring that nourishment reaches skin, hair, and nails. These are powerful polyphenols that can help reduce aging effects in the body— not only in skin but also with memory loss and heart disease.

Great levels of vitamins A, B-complex, C, and K, plus health-essential minerals copper, iron, potassium, and manganese, make black grapes the perfect superfood dessert choice, especially since they taste sweet and juicy, yet are very low in calories.

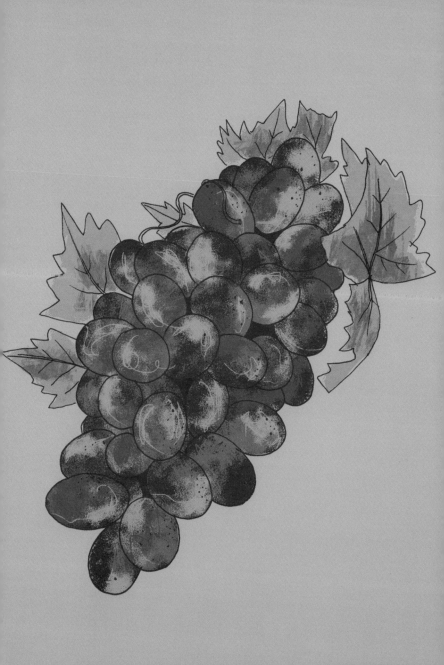

BLACK GRAPE AND RICOTTA SALAD

Inside: Treat yourself to this sweet
antiaging dessert.

You will need:

small bunch black grapes • 2 tablespoons ricotta • sea salt
• cinnamon • 1 tablespoon toasted hazelnuts • 2 squares
dark chocolate

To prepare:

Wash the black grapes and pat dry. Halve them and place in
a small dish. Place the ricotta in a small bowl, add a pinch of
sea salt and cinnamon, and mix well to combine, then spoon
over the black grape halves. Roughly chop the hazelnuts and
sprinkle them over the ricotta. Grate the dark chocolate over
the top to finish. Serve the salad chilled.

BLACK GRAPE TONER

Outside: Maximize the antioxidant benefits to your skin with this zesty treatment.

You will need:

small bunch black grapes • juice of ½ lemon • 4 tablespoons rose water or witch hazel • small glass jar with screw-top lid

To prepare:

Wash the black grapes and place in a blender with the lemon juice and rose water or witch hazel. Blend thoroughly, then strain the juice into the glass jar to remove the pulp.

To use:

Use a cotton ball to apply the treatment to your skin after cleansing. It will refresh and hydrate. Rose water is best for drier, more mature skin, while witch hazel is a good choice for younger or more oily skin.

BLUEBERRIES

One of the richest sources of disease-fighting antioxidants, blueberries are tiny powerhouses of important nutrients that keep mind and body in the very best of health.

The antioxidant power of blueberries combines with vitamins A, C, E, and K to offer protection from the free-radical damage that is responsible for premature skin aging and the development of some diseases, including cancer and diabetes. It also improves cell regeneration and strengthens capillaries, resulting in better skin tone and quality. High levels of anthocyanin—the compound that gives the blueberry its beautiful skin color—ensure clear and healthy eyes. Even brain power is boosted by a daily handful of these colorful superberries.

This fruit is high in fiber but, unlike many other fruits, low in sugar, making it the perfect healthy snack. Enjoy fresh, juicy berries during the summer months or reap the delicious benefits from frozen berries in winter. They are especially good in a smoothie or stirred through yogurt.

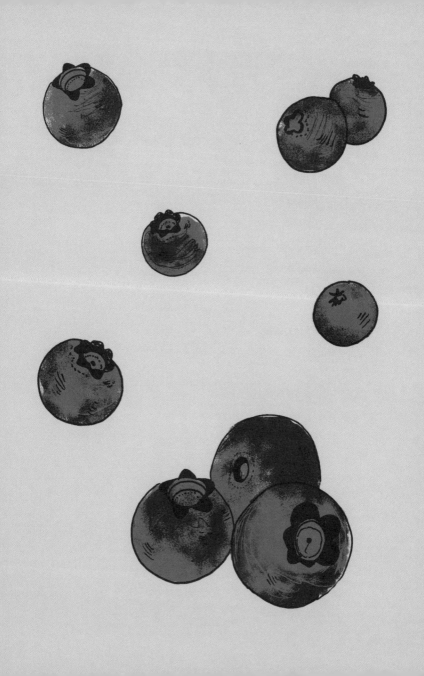

BLUEBERRY AND OAT COOKIES

Inside: Keep your skin looking youthful
with these berry-oaty treats.

You will need:

1 stick unsalted butter • 1 cup dark brown sugar • 1 egg
• 1 teaspoon vanilla extract • 1½ cups rolled oats • 1 cup
unrefined flour • ½ teaspoon baking powder • ½ teaspoon salt
• 2 teaspoons cinnamon • 1½ cups blueberries (fresh or frozen)

To prepare:

Preheat the oven to 350°F and line two baking sheets with
parchment paper. Cream the butter and sugar together
and add the beaten egg and vanilla extract. Stir in the oats,
flour, baking powder, salt, and cinnamon and combine
thoroughly. Gently fold in the blueberries.

Place spoonfuls of the mixture onto the baking sheets.
Bake for fifteen minutes until golden, then remove and cool
on wire racks.

BLUEBERRY EXFOLIATOR

Outside: Exfoliate, cleanse, and condition your skin with this berry-rich blend.

You will need:

¹/₃ cup blueberries • 1 teaspoon sugar • 1 tablespoon olive oil

• 1 tablespoon honey

To prepare:

In a small bowl, blend all the ingredients together until smooth.

To use:

Gently massage the exfoliator in circular strokes across your forehead, down your nose (taking care to avoid the eye area), across your cheeks, and around your chin. Rinse off with warm water and pat dry to reveal smooth, glowing skin. This exfoliator is great as a weekly treatment.

CHIA SEEDS

The power of this nutrient-packed, energy-boosting superseed
was recognized by the ancient Aztecs and Mayans. The word
chia meant "strength" to the Mayans and they would use the
seeds both as a medicine and as an everyday food.

Just one tablespoon of chia seeds, which are gluten-free, contains a
highly effective mix of vital vitamins and minerals, oils, protein, and
fiber, to keep the body and brain in peak condition. With high levels of
antioxidants and essential fatty acids—predominantly omega-3—chia
seeds help ensure skin, hair, and nails are well nourished. Impressive
levels of protein offer a good balance of essential amino acids for
healthy body function and the high fiber content helps to regulate
blood sugar levels and keep the digestive system running well.

Good levels of calcium, manganese, magnesium, phosphorus, zinc,
potassium, and B-complex vitamins simply add to this tiny seed's
power as the ultimate beauty weapon! Grown all year round in Mexico,
chia seeds can last up to two years without losing their nutritional
effectiveness—a great indication of their antioxidant power!

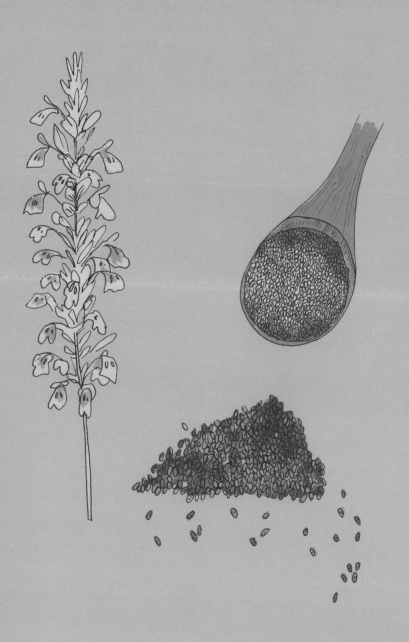

CHIA BREAKFAST SMOOTHIE

Inside: Give yourself a protein boost with this rich breakfast smoothie.

You will need:

1 ripe banana • 1 tablespoon chia seeds • 1 tablespoon peanut butter • 1 teaspoon honey • 1 cup whole milk • ground cinnamon

To prepare:

Chop the banana and place in a blender with the chia seeds, peanut butter, honey, and milk. Blend until rich and creamy and pour into a serving glass.

Sprinkle with cinnamon for a potassium-, calcium-, and protein-rich breakfast that will give you all the energy you need for a busy morning.

CHIA SKIN AND LIP OIL

Outside: Use this great winter treatment to
hydrate even the driest lips and skin.

You will need:

1 tablespoon chia seeds • 1 cup water • 1 teaspoon coconut oil

To prepare:

Place the chia seeds in a small glass bowl, cover with water,
and leave to soak overnight. The seeds will absorb the
water and form a gel-like substance. Add the coconut oil and
mix thoroughly.

To use:

Spread the treatment onto your face and lips. Leave on for
thirty minutes to moisturize. Your skin will glow with
radiance and your lips will be plump and smooth.

DATES

This superfood can be eaten fresh when in season—during fall—or all year round in its dried form. Dates are grown in the dry, arid conditions of Egypt and the Middle East and have a concentration of important vitamins and minerals—so much that many people believe that it is possible to survive for days in the desert with just water to drink and dates to eat.

A rich source of antioxidants, these sweet palm fruits are also high in calcium, iron, potassium, phosphorus, manganese, magnesium, and copper, all of which contribute to strong muscle development as well as healthy skin and hair. A high dietary fiber content helps regulate the digestive system, while promoting good bacteria in the intestines—and good digestion means improved absorption of nutrients from all foods. All in all, dates make a perfect, satisfying snack that leaves you glowing with health, inside and out.

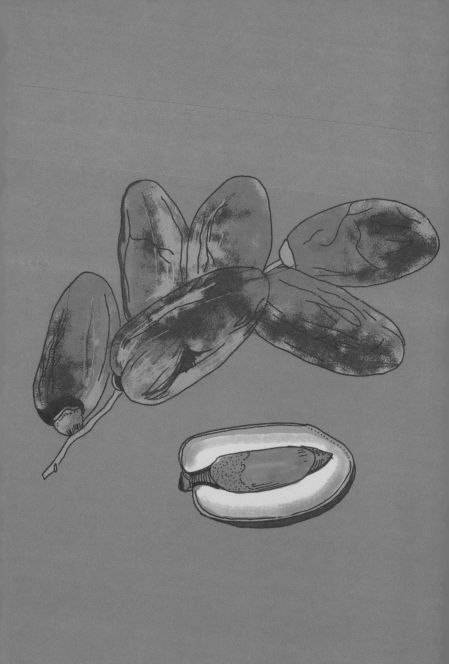

DATE AND BEET BLISS BALLS

Inside: Boost your muscle development with these mineral-rich delights.

You will need:

¾ cup dried dates • 1 cup almonds • 1 cup dried, shredded coconut • 1 cup finely grated beets • 1 tablespoon coconut oil • 1 teaspoon fresh ginger, finely chopped (optional) • Juice of ½ lemon

To prepare:

Remove the pits from the dates and place all the ingredients, except the lemon juice, in a food processor. Blend until the ingredients are finely processed and you have a soft, dough-like paste—if it's too solid, add a little lemon juice.

Taking a little of the mixture at a time, roll in your hands to form bite-sized balls. Place them on a baking sheet and refrigerate for fifteen minutes before eating.

DATE, YOGURT, AND HONEY FACE MASK

Outside: Cleanse and nourish your face for a radiant and youthful complexion.

You will need:

4 dried dates • 1 cup warm water • 1 tablespoon Greek yogurt

• 1 teaspoon honey

To prepare:

Remove the pits from the dates and soak the flesh in warm water for one hour. Drain, and place in a blender, along with the yogurt and honey. Blend together until smooth.

To use:

Gently massage the face mask onto your face, right up to the eyes and down the neck. Leave for fifteen minutes, before rinsing off with warm water to reveal softer, refreshed, and healthier-looking skin.

OLIVES

Juicy green or rich black olives have long been considered a health-promoting food throughout the Mediterranean. Ripe and ready for harvest during the summer months, they are rich in antioxidants, important minerals and vitamins, good omega-6 and omega-3 oils, and phytosterols, which are great for helping reduce cholesterol and keeping your heart healthy. Rich in skin-loving vitamin E and carotenoids, olives also help protect against inflammation and keep the nervous system healthy.

Olives contain good quantities of calcium, manganese, iron, copper, and zinc, as well as essential B-complex vitamins, all of which contribute to smooth, supple skin, and shiny hair. Cold-pressed virgin olive oil is the best to use in salad dressings: not only does this have optimum nutritional value, it also has the best taste!

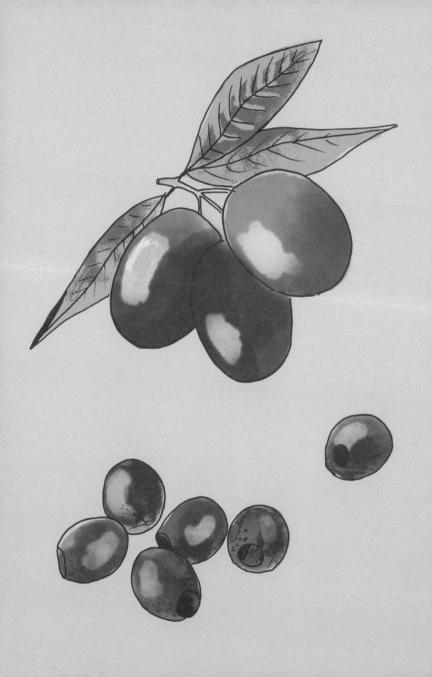

MARINATED OLIVES WITH FETA

Inside: Boost your heart health with
this phytosterol-rich dish.

You will need:

½ cup pitted black olives • 7 oz feta cheese • sprig of
rosemary • juice of ½ lemon • 1 tablespoon olive oil • sea salt
• black pepper

To prepare:

Chop the olives, dice the feta, and place both in a small serving
bowl. Chop the rosemary leaves and add to the bowl, along
with the lemon juice and the olive oil. Dust with sea salt and
black pepper and leave the flavors to infuse for thirty
minutes. Serve on crackers or toasted sourdough bread.

OLIVE OIL HAIR TREATMENT

Outside: Apply this deep-reaching, vitamin-E-rich
oil for softer, glossier hair.

You will need:

1 egg yolk • 2 tablespoons olive oil • 1 teaspoon lemon juice

To prepare:

Beat the egg yolk in a small bowl, then add the olive oil and
lemon juice and combine thoroughly.

To use:

Massage the mixture into dry hair, taking care to include
the ends. Leave for fifteen minutes, then rinse in warm water,
and shampoo and condition as usual. The result? Shiny,
supersoft hair.

SEAWEED

There are many types of edible seaweed available, including kelp, spirulina, and red and brown algae. Although these seaweeds are popular and available as dried powders for mixing into smoothies or sprinkling over salads and soups, the most easily available seaweed is nori, which can be bought dried and in sheets.

Seaweed is rich in chlorophyll, a great natural detoxifier and alkalizer of the blood. It is also a welcome source of vitamin K, which is important for healthy blood formation. Seaweed's high iodine content ensures optimum functioning of the thyroid gland, which produces the essential hormones for all the body's cells in addition to regulating the metabolism. Other valuable nutrients include vitamins A and B12, omega-3 essential fatty acids, and a high level of calcium, all of which contribute to healthy skin, hair, and nails.

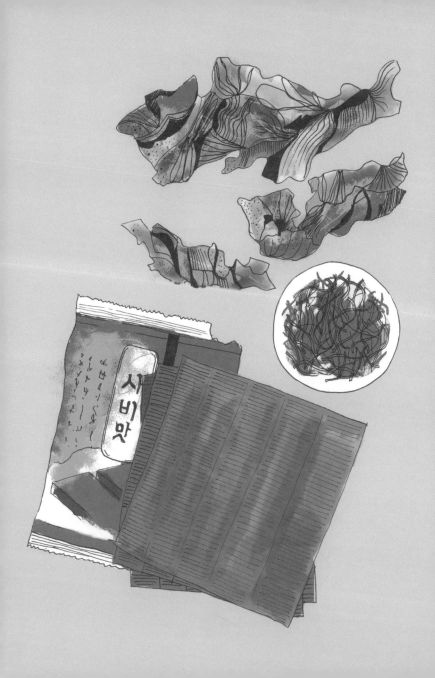

NORI WRAPS

Inside: Make these chlorophyll-rich wraps
for a cleansing, alkalizing boost.

You will need:

½ ripe avocado • juice of ½ lemon • sea salt • black pepper
• 1 carrot • 3 dried nori sheets • chili flakes • 3 cooked
asparagus spears • 1 handful spinach leaves

To prepare:

Mash the avocado with the lemon juice and add sea salt and
black pepper to taste. Peel the carrot and cut into thin
julienned sticks. Lay out the nori sheets, spread each with
avocado, and sprinkle with chili flakes.

Layer the carrot sticks, asparagus spears, and spinach leaves
along one edge of each nori sheet, then roll to form the wrap.
Serve immediately.

SEAWEED FACE MASK

Outside: Try this powerful hydration boost
for a youthful complexion.

You will need:

2 nori sheets • 1 cup freshly boiled water

To prepare:

This is the simplest of all homemade beauty treatments! Allow
the boiled water to cool. While still warm, pour the water over
the nori sheets and leave until softened.

To use:

Break small sections off the nori sheets and apply all over
your face, pressing into your skin. Avoid the eye area. Close
your eyes and relax for twenty minutes. Remove the seaweed
using a washcloth and rinse your skin in warm water. Pat dry
to reveal soft and glowing skin.

INDEX